The Student's Handbook on Bacterial Infectious Diseases: Causes, Symptoms, and Treatments

ROBERT

The Student's Handbook on Bacterial Infectious Diseases: Causes, Symptoms, and Treatments

Copyright © 2023 by ROBERT

All rights reserved. No part of this book may be reproduced or transmitted in any form or by any means, electronic or mechanical, including photocopying, recording, or by any information storage and retrieval system, without permission in writing from the publisher.

This book is a work of fiction. Names, characters, places, and incidents either are the product of the author's imagination or are used fictitiously. Any resemblance to actual events, locales, persons, living or dead, is entirely coincidental.

The first edition was published in 2023

ISBN:
Published by:
Sunshine
1663 Liberty Drive
Hyderabad, IN 47403
www.Sunshinepublishers.com

This book is self-published using on-demand printing and publishing, which allows it to be printed and distributed globally

TABLE OF CONTENT

Chapter 1: Introduction to Bacterial Infectious Diseases — 07

Understanding Bacterial Infections

Importance of Studying Bacterial Infectious Diseases

Chapter 2: Basics of Bacteria — 11

Classification of Bacteria

Structure and Function of Bacteria

Reproduction and Life Cycle of Bacteria

Chapter 3: Common Bacterial Infectious Diseases — 17

Tuberculosis

Staphylococcal Infections

Streptococcal Infections

Cholera

Salmonella Infections

Chapter 4: Causes and Transmission of Bacterial Infectious Diseases 27

Routes of Transmission

Factors Contributing to Bacterial Infections

Nosocomial Infections

Chapter 5: Symptoms and Diagnosis of Bacterial Infectious Diseases 33

General Symptoms of Bacterial Infections

Diagnostic Methods for Bacterial Infections

Laboratory Tests for Bacterial Infections

Chapter 6: Treatment and Management of Bacterial Infectious Diseases 39

Antibiotics and their Role in Treating Bacterial Infections

Vaccines for Bacterial Infections

Prevention Strategies for Bacterial Infections

Chapter 7: Antibiotic Resistance in Bacterial Infectious Diseases   45

Understanding Antibiotic Resistance

Factors Contributing to Antibiotic Resistance

Impact of Antibiotic Resistance on Bacterial Infections

Chapter 8: Emerging Bacterial Infectious Diseases   51

Methicillin-Resistant Staphylococcus aureus (MRSA)

Clostridioides difficile Infections

Carbapenem-Resistant Enterobacteriaceae (CRE)

Chapter 9: Case Studies: Real-Life Examples of Bacterial Infectious Diseases   57

Tuberculosis Outbreak in a Community

Contamination of Food with Salmonella

Hospital-Acquired Infections: Case of MRSA

Chapter 10: Future Perspectives in Bacterial Infectious Diseases 63

Advancements in Bacterial Infection Research

Potential Solutions for Antibiotic Resistance

Importance of Public Health Education and Awareness

Chapter 11: Conclusion and Resources 69

Summary of Key Points

Additional Resources for Further Reading

Glossary of Terms

Chapter 1: Introduction to Bacterial Infectious Diseases

Understanding Bacterial Infections

Bacterial infections are a common occurrence in our daily lives, and it is crucial for students to have a fundamental understanding of these infectious diseases. In this subchapter, we will delve into the causes, symptoms, and treatments of bacterial infections, equipping students with the knowledge necessary to protect themselves and others from these harmful microorganisms.

Causes:
Bacterial infections are caused by the invasion and multiplication of bacteria within the human body. Bacteria can enter the body through various means, including direct contact with an infected person, ingestion of contaminated food or water, or through the air we breathe. Understanding the modes of transmission is essential in preventing the spread of bacterial infections.

Symptoms:
The symptoms of bacterial infections can vary depending on the type of bacteria involved and the affected body part. Common symptoms include fever, fatigue, coughing, sneezing, sore throat, diarrhea, and skin rashes. It is important for students to be aware of these symptoms to seek timely medical attention and prevent the infection from worsening.

Treatments:
Treating bacterial infections often involves the use of antibiotics, which are medications specifically designed to kill or inhibit the growth of bacteria. However, it is crucial to note

that not all bacterial infections require antibiotics, and their misuse can lead to antibiotic resistance. Students will learn about the importance of completing the full course of antibiotics as prescribed by a healthcare professional and the significance of using antibiotics judiciously.

Prevention:
Prevention is always better than cure, and students will be educated on various preventive measures to reduce the risk of bacterial infections. These preventive measures include practicing good personal hygiene, such as frequent handwashing with soap and water, avoiding close contact with infected individuals, maintaining a clean environment, and following proper food safety practices.

Understanding bacterial infections is essential for students interested in the field of infectious diseases. By acquiring knowledge about the causes, symptoms, treatments, and preventive measures, students can protect themselves and contribute to the overall well-being of their communities. This subchapter will serve as a valuable resource for students, equipping them with the necessary tools to combat bacterial infections and promote a healthier society.

Importance of Studying Bacterial Infectious Diseases

The importance of studying bacterial infectious diseases cannot be overstated, especially for students interested in the field of infectious diseases. Bacterial infections have been a significant threat to human health throughout history, and understanding these diseases is crucial for their prevention, diagnosis, and treatment.

One of the primary reasons for studying bacterial infectious diseases is the potential public health impact. Bacteria can cause a wide range of infections, from mild illnesses to life-threatening conditions. By studying these diseases, students can learn about the various bacteria responsible for infections and the mechanisms by which they spread. This knowledge is essential for developing effective public health strategies, such as vaccination programs, hygiene practices, and infection control measures.

Moreover, studying bacterial infectious diseases helps students understand the symptoms and clinical manifestations associated with these infections. Recognizing the signs of bacterial infections is vital for early diagnosis and appropriate treatment. This knowledge can save lives and prevent the progression of diseases to severe stages.

In addition, learning about bacterial infectious diseases provides students with an understanding of antibiotic resistance. Overuse and misuse of antibiotics have led to the emergence of drug-resistant bacteria, posing a significant global health challenge. By studying these diseases, students can gain insights into the factors contributing to antibiotic resistance and their implications for treatment. This knowledge is crucial in promoting responsible antibiotic use and developing alternative treatment strategies.

Furthermore, studying bacterial infectious diseases allows students to explore the latest advancements in diagnostic techniques and treatment options. The field of infectious diseases is rapidly evolving, with new technologies and therapies being developed. By staying updated with these advancements, students can contribute to the field and help improve patient outcomes.

Lastly, studying bacterial infectious diseases offers exciting career opportunities. With a solid understanding of these diseases, students can pursue careers as clinical microbiologists, epidemiologists, infectious disease specialists, or public health professionals. The demand for experts in this field is high, making it a rewarding and fulfilling career path.

In conclusion, the study of bacterial infectious diseases is of utmost importance for students interested in the field of infectious diseases. It provides a foundation for public health strategies, improves diagnostic and treatment approaches, and offers promising career opportunities. By understanding these diseases, students can contribute to the prevention, control, and management of bacterial infections, ultimately benefiting global health.

Chapter 2: Basics of Bacteria

Classification of Bacteria

Bacteria are microscopic organisms that play a crucial role in the world of infectious diseases. Understanding the classification of bacteria is essential for students studying infectious diseases. This subchapter will delve into the various ways bacteria can be classified, providing students with a comprehensive understanding of these microscopic organisms.

The classification of bacteria is primarily based on their morphological, physiological, and genetic characteristics. Morphological classification involves examining the shape, arrangement, and structure of bacterial cells. Bacteria can be classified into three main shapes: cocci (spherical), bacilli (rod-shaped), and spirilla (spiral-shaped). The arrangement of these cells can further classify bacteria into clusters, chains, or pairs.

Physiological classification focuses on the bacteria's metabolic capabilities and growth requirements. Bacteria can be classified based on their oxygen requirements, such as aerobic bacteria that require oxygen for growth, anaerobic bacteria that cannot tolerate oxygen, and facultative anaerobes that can grow with or without oxygen. This classification is important as it helps students understand the environmental conditions in which bacteria thrive and cause infections.

Genetic classification, also known as molecular classification, relies on the analysis of bacterial DNA. This classification method has revolutionized our understanding of bacterial diversity and relatedness. Bacteria can be classified based on their genetic similarities, allowing scientists to identify specific strains responsible for infectious diseases. This knowledge is crucial for developing targeted treatments and prevention strategies.

Furthermore, bacteria can also be classified based on their Gram staining properties. The Gram stain is a technique used to differentiate bacteria into two groups: Gram-positive and Gram-negative. This classification is particularly important as it helps determine the appropriate antibiotic treatment for bacterial infections.

Understanding the classification of bacteria is vital for students studying infectious diseases. It enables them to identify and categorize different bacterial species, aiding in the diagnosis and treatment of bacterial infections. By knowing the morphological, physiological, and genetic characteristics of bacteria, students can gain insights into their pathogenicity and develop effective strategies to combat bacterial infections.

In conclusion, the classification of bacteria plays a fundamental role in understanding infectious diseases. It allows students to categorize bacteria based on their morphology, physiology, genetics, and staining properties. This knowledge enables the identification of specific bacterial strains responsible for infections, leading to more effective treatments and prevention strategies. By studying the classification of bacteria, students can contribute to the field of infectious diseases and make significant advancements in combating these microscopic organisms.

Structure and Function of Bacteria

Bacteria are single-celled microorganisms that play a significant role in infectious diseases. Understanding their structure and function is crucial for students studying infectious diseases. This subchapter will delve into the intricate details of bacterial structure and how it relates to their function in causing diseases.

The structure of bacteria is relatively simple compared to other organisms. They consist of a cell membrane, cytoplasm, genetic material, and a cell wall. Some bacteria also possess additional structures such as flagella, pili, and capsules, which aid in their survival and pathogenicity.

The cell membrane is a vital component of bacteria as it controls the movement of substances in and out of the cell. It also houses various proteins that facilitate important cellular functions. The cytoplasm, on the other hand, contains enzymes, nutrients, and other molecules necessary for bacterial metabolism and growth.

The genetic material of bacteria is located in the form of a single circular DNA molecule within the cytoplasm. This DNA contains the instructions for bacterial replication, as well as the genes responsible for producing virulence factors that enable bacteria to cause diseases.

The cell wall, a rigid structure surrounding the cell membrane, provides shape, support, and protection to bacteria. It is composed of peptidoglycan, a unique molecule found only in bacterial cell walls. The presence or absence of this molecule determines whether bacteria are categorized as Gram-positive or Gram-negative, a crucial distinction in diagnosing and treating bacterial infections.

Flagella, which are whip-like structures, allow bacteria to move in liquid environments. Pili are hair-like projections that enable bacteria to adhere to surfaces, including host tissues, promoting colonization and subsequent infection. Capsules, a slimy layer surrounding some bacteria, protect them from immune responses and antibiotics, enhancing their ability to cause disease.

Understanding the structure and function of bacteria is essential for studying infectious diseases. By unraveling the mechanisms by which bacteria interact with their environment and host organisms, scientists can develop effective treatments and preventive strategies. Additionally, knowledge of bacterial structure and function helps identify specific targets for drug development and vaccination.

In conclusion, bacteria possess a relatively simple yet highly efficient structure that enables them to cause infectious diseases. Their cell membrane, cytoplasm, genetic material, and cell wall, along with additional structures such as flagella, pili, and capsules, all contribute to their pathogenicity. Students studying infectious diseases must grasp the intricacies of bacterial structure and function to comprehend the underlying mechanisms of bacterial infections and devise effective treatment strategies.

Reproduction and Life Cycle of Bacteria

In the fascinating world of microbiology, the reproduction and life cycle of bacteria play a crucial role in understanding the causes, symptoms, and treatments of infectious diseases. Bacteria, being single-celled organisms, have a unique and efficient way of multiplying and spreading, making them a significant threat to human health. In this subchapter, we will delve into the intricacies of bacterial reproduction and explore how it contributes to the development and transmission of infectious diseases.

Bacteria reproduce through a process called binary fission, in which a single bacterial cell divides into two identical daughter cells. This rapid division allows bacteria to multiply exponentially, leading to the formation of colonies within a short period. However, it is important to note that bacterial reproduction is not always a smooth process. Various factors such as nutrient availability, temperature, pH levels, and the presence of antibiotics can influence the rate of reproduction.

The life cycle of bacteria involves several stages, starting with the lag phase, where bacteria adapt to the new environment and prepare for reproduction. This is followed by the exponential growth phase, where bacteria multiply rapidly, leading to a substantial increase in population size. As resources become limited, the growth rate slows down, and bacteria enter the stationary phase. In this phase, the number of bacterial cells produced is balanced by the number of cells dying or becoming dormant. Finally, the decline phase occurs when the bacteria can no longer sustain themselves due to resource depletion or other adverse conditions.

Understanding the life cycle of bacteria is vital in the study of infectious diseases. It helps us comprehend how bacteria can rapidly spread and cause infections within a short period. Bacteria can be transmitted through various means, including direct contact, airborne particles, contaminated food or water, and insect vectors. By understanding their life cycle, we can identify potential points of intervention to prevent the transmission and spread of these diseases.

Moreover, studying the reproduction and life cycle of bacteria provides insight into the development of effective treatments. Antibiotics, for instance, target specific stages of the bacterial life cycle to inhibit reproduction or kill bacteria. By interrupting the reproduction process, we can prevent the spread of infectious diseases and aid in the recovery of infected individuals.

In conclusion, the reproduction and life cycle of bacteria are fundamental concepts in understanding infectious diseases. By unraveling the intricacies of bacterial reproduction, we gain valuable knowledge that helps us develop strategies for prevention, control, and treatment. As students delving into the world of infectious diseases, it is crucial to grasp these concepts to contribute to the fight against bacterial infections and improve global health.

Chapter 3: Common Bacterial Infectious Diseases

Tuberculosis

Tuberculosis, also known as TB, is a bacterial infectious disease that primarily affects the lungs but can also spread to other parts of the body. It is caused by Mycobacterium tuberculosis, a bacterium that is transmitted through the air when an infected person coughs or sneezes. This makes TB highly contagious and poses a significant public health concern.

Students studying infectious diseases need to be aware of tuberculosis due to its global impact and the challenges it presents in terms of diagnosis, treatment, and prevention. In this subchapter, we will explore the causes, symptoms, and treatments of tuberculosis.

Causes: As mentioned earlier, TB is caused by the bacterium Mycobacterium tuberculosis. It is primarily transmitted through respiratory droplets when an infected person coughs, sneezes, or talks. Factors that increase the risk of contracting TB include close contact with an infected individual, living in crowded conditions, having a weakened immune system (such as in HIV/AIDS patients), and malnutrition.

Symptoms: The symptoms of tuberculosis can vary depending on the stage of the disease. Common symptoms include persistent cough (lasting more than three weeks), chest pain, coughing up blood, fatigue, weight loss, night sweats, and fever. In some cases, TB can also affect other organs such as the kidneys, spine, or brain, leading to specific symptoms related to those areas.

Treatment: Tuberculosis is a treatable and curable disease. The standard treatment for TB involves a combination of antibiotics taken over a specific period, typically six to nine months. It is crucial to complete the entire course of medication to prevent drug resistance. Directly Observed Therapy (DOT) is often used to ensure adherence to the treatment regimen. In some cases, drug-resistant strains of TB may require additional or alternative medications, which can be more challenging to treat.

Prevention: To prevent the spread of tuberculosis, it is essential to practice good respiratory hygiene, such as covering the mouth and nose when coughing or sneezing. Adequate ventilation in living and working spaces can also help reduce the risk of transmission. Vaccination with the Bacillus Calmette-Guérin (BCG) vaccine is available and recommended in countries with a high burden of TB.

In conclusion, tuberculosis is a significant global health concern, and students studying infectious diseases should be well-informed about its causes, symptoms, and treatments. By understanding the risk factors and adopting preventive measures, we can contribute to the control and eventual eradication of this infectious disease.

Staphylococcal Infections

Staphylococcal infections are a common type of bacterial infection caused by Staphylococcus bacteria. These infections can range from mild to severe and can affect various parts of the body, including the skin, respiratory tract, and bloodstream. In this subchapter, we will explore the causes, symptoms, and treatments of staphylococcal infections, providing valuable information for students interested in the field of infectious diseases.

Causes:
Staphylococcal infections are primarily caused by the bacteria Staphylococcus aureus, commonly found on the skin or in the nose of healthy individuals. However, these bacteria can become harmful when they enter the body through cuts, wounds, or other open areas. Factors such as poor hygiene, weakened immune system, and close contact with infected individuals can increase the risk of developing a staphylococcal infection.

Symptoms:
The symptoms of staphylococcal infections vary depending on the affected area. Skin infections typically present as red, swollen, and painful sores or boils filled with pus. These can be accompanied by fever and fatigue. In more severe cases, staph infections can lead to pneumonia, bloodstream infections, or toxic shock syndrome, which may cause symptoms like high fever, difficulty breathing, and confusion.

Treatments:
Treatment for staphylococcal infections usually involves antibiotics that target the specific strain of Staphylococcus bacteria causing the infection. It is important to complete the

full course of antibiotics as prescribed by a healthcare professional to effectively eliminate the bacteria. In cases of skin infections, draining the abscess or infected area may be necessary. Proper wound care, good hygiene practices, and avoiding close contact with infected individuals can help prevent the spread of staph infections.

Prevention:
Preventing staphylococcal infections involves practicing good hygiene, such as regular handwashing with soap and water. It is also crucial to keep wounds clean and covered until they heal completely. Avoiding sharing personal items, such as towels or razors, can minimize the risk of transmission. In healthcare settings, strict adherence to infection control measures, including proper sterilization of medical equipment, is essential to prevent the spread of staph infections.

In conclusion, staphylococcal infections are a common type of bacterial infection caused by Staphylococcus bacteria. Understanding the causes, symptoms, and treatments of these infections is crucial for students interested in the field of infectious diseases. By promoting good hygiene practices and implementing appropriate preventive measures, we can effectively reduce the incidence and impact of staphylococcal infections in our communities.

Streptococcal Infections

Streptococcal infections are a group of bacterial infections caused by the Streptococcus bacteria. These infections can range from mild to severe and can affect various parts of the body, including the throat, skin, and respiratory system. As students interested in infectious diseases, it is crucial to understand the causes, symptoms, and treatments of streptococcal infections to protect ourselves and others from these potentially harmful bacteria.

One of the most common types of streptococcal infections is strep throat. It is highly contagious and spreads through respiratory droplets when an infected person coughs or sneezes. Symptoms of strep throat include a sore throat, difficulty swallowing, swollen lymph nodes, and fever. If left untreated, it can lead to complications such as rheumatic fever or kidney inflammation.

Another type of streptococcal infection is cellulitis, which affects the skin and underlying tissues. It usually occurs when the bacteria enter through a cut or wound. Symptoms include redness, swelling, warmth, and pain in the affected area. Cellulitis can be severe and may require hospitalization if not treated promptly.

Invasive streptococcal infections, such as necrotizing fasciitis or streptococcal toxic shock syndrome, are rare but life-threatening. These infections occur when the bacteria invade deeper tissues and spread rapidly. Symptoms include severe pain, fever, swelling, and a rapidly spreading rash. Immediate medical attention is crucial in these cases.

Treatment for streptococcal infections typically involves antibiotics to kill the bacteria. It is essential to complete the full course of antibiotics prescribed by the healthcare provider to ensure complete eradication of the bacteria and prevent recurrence or antibiotic resistance. Pain relievers and fever reducers may also be recommended to alleviate symptoms.

Preventing streptococcal infections involves practicing good hygiene, such as washing hands frequently, covering the mouth and nose when coughing or sneezing, and avoiding close contact with infected individuals. It is also crucial to avoid sharing personal items like utensils or towels, which can spread the bacteria.

In conclusion, streptococcal infections are a group of bacterial infections caused by the Streptococcus bacteria. As students interested in infectious diseases, it is vital to be aware of the causes, symptoms, and treatments of streptococcal infections. By practicing good hygiene and seeking prompt medical attention, we can protect ourselves and others from these potentially harmful bacteria.

Cholera

Cholera: A Devastating Bacterial Infection

Introduction:
Cholera, a highly contagious bacterial infection, has plagued humanity for centuries. It is essential for students studying infectious diseases to have a comprehensive understanding of this disease, as it continues to pose a significant threat in certain parts of the world. This subchapter will provide an overview of cholera, including its causes, symptoms, and treatments.

Causes:
Cholera is caused by the bacterium Vibrio cholerae, which thrives in contaminated water and food sources. The primary mode of transmission occurs through the consumption of contaminated water or food, especially in areas lacking proper sanitation facilities. This bacterium can survive in harsh environments, making it particularly resilient and capable of causing devastating outbreaks.

Symptoms:
The symptoms of cholera can range from mild to severe, with the latter often leading to life-threatening dehydration. Common symptoms include profuse diarrhea, vomiting, and abdominal cramps. Affected individuals may rapidly lose fluids, leading to extreme thirst, dry mouth, sunken eyes, and reduced urine output. If left untreated, cholera can cause severe electrolyte imbalances, muscle cramps, and shock.

Treatment:
Prompt treatment is crucial in managing cholera cases. Oral rehydration therapy (ORT) is the cornerstone of treatment, as

it helps replenish the lost fluids and electrolytes. This simple, cost-effective solution involves administering a mixture of clean water, salt, and sugar. In severe cases, intravenous fluids may be necessary to restore fluid balance.

Prevention:
Preventing the spread of cholera requires a multi-faceted approach. Access to clean water and improved sanitation facilities is crucial in reducing the risk of contamination. Educating communities about proper hygiene practices, such as handwashing, is also essential. Vaccination against cholera is available in some regions and can be effective in certain situations.

Global Impact:
Cholera continues to heavily impact certain regions, particularly those with limited access to clean water and proper sanitation. Outbreaks often occur after natural disasters or in crowded, unsanitary conditions, such as refugee camps. Understanding the global impact of cholera is vital for students studying infectious diseases, as it highlights the importance of implementing preventative measures and providing timely medical interventions.

Conclusion:
Cholera remains a significant health concern in many parts of the world, emphasizing the need for continued research, prevention, and treatment efforts. Students studying infectious diseases should grasp the causes, symptoms, and treatments associated with cholera to contribute to the global fight against this devastating bacterial infection. By combining knowledge with action, we can work towards a future where cholera is no longer a threat to human health.

Salmonella Infections

Salmonella infections are a type of bacterial infection caused by the Salmonella bacteria. These bacteria are commonly found in the intestines of animals, including poultry, cattle, and reptiles. Salmonella is a leading cause of foodborne illness worldwide, and it can be transmitted to humans through the consumption of contaminated food or water.

Symptoms of Salmonella infections typically appear within 12 to 72 hours after exposure and may include diarrhea, abdominal cramps, fever, and vomiting. In some cases, the infection may become severe and require hospitalization. It is important to seek medical attention if you experience these symptoms, as prompt treatment can help alleviate the severity and duration of the illness.

Preventing Salmonella infections starts with proper food handling and hygiene practices. Always wash your hands thoroughly with soap and water before and after handling food, especially raw meats and eggs. Cook food, particularly poultry and eggs, to an appropriate internal temperature to kill any bacteria present. Avoid consuming raw eggs or undercooked meats, as they can be potential sources of Salmonella contamination.

Additionally, it is crucial to practice good kitchen hygiene by keeping surfaces clean and using separate cutting boards for raw meats and fresh produce. Refrigerate perishable foods promptly and discard any food that has been left at room temperature for more than two hours. By following these simple guidelines, you can significantly reduce your risk of contracting a Salmonella infection.

If you suspect that you have a Salmonella infection, it is important to consult a healthcare professional. Your doctor may order a stool sample to confirm the diagnosis. In most cases, Salmonella infections resolve on their own within a week without specific treatment. However, it is essential to stay hydrated by drinking plenty of fluids to prevent dehydration caused by diarrhea.

In rare cases, Salmonella infections can lead to complications, especially in individuals with weakened immune systems, such as the elderly, infants, and those with chronic illnesses. These complications may include bloodstream infections, which require immediate medical attention.

By understanding the causes, symptoms, and preventive measures of Salmonella infections, you can protect yourself and others from this common bacterial illness. Remember to prioritize food safety and personal hygiene to reduce the risk of contamination and promote a healthy lifestyle.

Chapter 4: Causes and Transmission of Bacterial Infectious Diseases

Routes of Transmission

Understanding how bacterial infectious diseases are transmitted is crucial in preventing their spread. Bacterial infections can be transmitted through various routes, and recognizing these routes can help students take necessary precautions to protect themselves and others. This subchapter explores the different routes of transmission to raise awareness and promote responsible actions among students.

1. Direct Contact: Bacterial infections can spread through direct contact with infected individuals. This can occur through physical contact, such as shaking hands or hugging, or through activities like sexual intercourse. It is important to be cautious and practice good hygiene to prevent the transmission of bacteria.

2. Indirect Contact: Bacteria can also be transmitted indirectly through contaminated objects or surfaces. For example, touching doorknobs, sharing utensils, or using uncleaned gym equipment can all contribute to the spread of bactcria. Regular handwashing and proper sanitization can significantly reduce the risk of transmission.

3. Respiratory Droplets: Many bacterial infections are spread through respiratory droplets expelled when an infected person coughs or sneezes. These droplets can be inhaled by others in close proximity, leading to infection. Maintaining proper respiratory hygiene, such as covering the mouth and nose while coughing or sneezing, can help prevent the spread of bacteria.

4. Food and Water: Contaminated food and water can be a source of bacterial infections. Consumption of undercooked or improperly stored food, as well as drinking contaminated water, can introduce harmful bacteria into the body. Students should be mindful of food safety practices and ensure they drink clean and treated water.

5. Vector-Borne Transmission: Some bacterial diseases are transmitted through vectors such as mosquitoes, ticks, or fleas. These vectors act as carriers, transferring bacteria from infected animals to humans. Understanding the regions and seasons when vector activity is high can help students take necessary precautions, such as using insect repellents or wearing protective clothing.

By understanding the routes of transmission, students can actively take steps to minimize their risk of bacterial infections. Practicing good hygiene, such as regular handwashing, covering the mouth and nose while coughing or sneezing, and maintaining cleanliness in personal and shared spaces, can greatly reduce the spread of bacteria. Additionally, being aware of the risks associated with contaminated food, water, and vectors can help students make informed choices to protect themselves and others.

Remember, knowledge is power when it comes to bacterial infectious diseases. By staying informed and taking appropriate preventive measures, students can play an essential role in minimizing the impact of these diseases on their own health and the health of their communities. Stay vigilant, stay informed, and stay healthy!

Factors Contributing to Bacterial Infections

In order to understand bacterial infections and their impact on human health, it is crucial to explore the various factors that contribute to their occurrence. Bacterial infections can affect anyone, regardless of age or gender, and understanding the underlying causes can help students take preventative measures and make informed decisions about their health. This subchapter aims to shed light on the key factors that contribute to bacterial infections.

1. Poor Personal Hygiene: One of the primary factors contributing to bacterial infections is poor personal hygiene. Insufficient handwashing, not covering the mouth while coughing or sneezing, and neglecting to clean and sanitize personal belongings can all increase the risk of bacterial transmission.

2. Contaminated Food and Water: Consuming contaminated food or water can introduce harmful bacteria into the body. Inadequate cooking, improper storage, and exposure to unclean water sources are common ways in which bacteria can enter the human system.

3. Weakened Immune System: Individuals with weakened immune systems are more susceptible to bacterial infections. Factors such as stress, lack of sleep, poor nutrition, chronic diseases, and certain medications can compromise the body's ability to fight off bacteria effectively.

4. Close Contact with Infected Individuals: Bacterial infections are highly contagious and can spread through close contact with infected individuals. This includes direct contact, sharing

personal items, and being in close proximity to someone who is sick.

5. Environmental Factors: Certain environmental conditions can contribute to the growth and spread of bacteria. For example, warm and humid environments provide an ideal breeding ground for bacteria, increasing the risk of infections.

6. Healthcare-Associated Infections: Healthcare facilities can harbor bacteria that can cause infections. Factors such as inadequate sterilization of medical equipment, improper hand hygiene among healthcare workers, and the presence of antibiotic-resistant bacteria in hospitals contribute to healthcare-associated infections.

7. Poor Vaccination Coverage: Vaccinations play a crucial role in preventing bacterial infections. Low vaccination coverage can lead to outbreaks and an increased risk of infection among the population.

By understanding these factors, students can take proactive steps to minimize their risk of bacterial infections. Practicing good personal hygiene, ensuring food and water safety, maintaining a healthy lifestyle, and staying up-to-date with vaccinations are all effective strategies for preventing bacterial infections. Additionally, promoting awareness about these factors among peers and communities can contribute to the overall prevention and control of bacterial infectious diseases.

Nosocomial Infections

In a healthcare setting, the last thing one would expect is to contract an infection. Unfortunately, nosocomial infections, also known as healthcare-associated infections (HAIs), are a significant concern for patients and healthcare providers alike. This subchapter will delve into the causes, symptoms, and treatments of nosocomial infections, with a focus on bacteria-related diseases.

Nosocomial infections are infections that are acquired during a hospital stay or any healthcare-related procedure. These infections can be caused by a range of bacteria, including Staphylococcus aureus, Escherichia coli, and Pseudomonas aeruginosa, among others. The transmission of these bacteria can occur through various means, such as direct contact with healthcare providers, contaminated medical devices, or exposure to unclean surfaces.

Symptoms of nosocomial infections can vary depending on the type of bacteria involved and the site of infection. Common signs include fever, wound infections, urinary tract infections, pneumonia, and bloodstream infections. It is crucial for students to recognize these symptoms, as early detection can lead to prompt treatment and better patient outcomes.

Prevention is key in combating nosocomial infections. Students should familiarize themselves with proper hand hygiene techniques, including regular handwashing and the use of hand sanitizers. Additionally, they should adhere to infection control protocols, such as wearing personal protective equipment (PPE) when necessary and properly disinfecting medical equipment.

When it comes to treatment, healthcare providers may prescribe antibiotics based on the specific bacteria causing the infection. However, it is important to note that overuse or misuse of antibiotics can contribute to the development of antibiotic-resistant bacteria, which poses a significant threat to global health. Students should be aware of this issue and understand the importance of using antibiotics judiciously.

Furthermore, students must also be aware of their role in advocating for patient safety. By being vigilant, they can help identify potential breaches in infection control practices and report them promptly to the appropriate authorities.

In conclusion, nosocomial infections are a serious concern within the realm of infectious diseases. Students must educate themselves about the causes, symptoms, and treatments of these infections to protect themselves and others. By following proper hygiene practices and infection control protocols, students can play an active role in preventing the spread of nosocomial infections and ensuring safer healthcare environments for all.

Chapter 5: Symptoms and Diagnosis of Bacterial Infectious Diseases

General Symptoms of Bacterial Infections

When it comes to bacterial infections, understanding the general symptoms can help you recognize and seek appropriate medical attention in a timely manner. Bacterial infections are caused by harmful bacteria invading the body and disrupting its normal functions. As students interested in infectious diseases, it is crucial to be aware of these symptoms, as they can vary depending on the type of infection and the affected body system.

One of the most common symptoms of a bacterial infection is fever, which is the body's natural response to fighting off harmful bacteria. Fever is often accompanied by chills, excessive sweating, and general malaise. Additionally, you may experience fatigue and a lack of energy, as your body works hard to combat the infection.

Another telltale sign of a bacterial infection is inflammation. This can manifest as redness, swelling, and pain in the affected area. For example, if the infection is in the respiratory system, you may experience a sore throat, coughing, and difficulty breathing. Similarly, a bacterial skin infection may cause redness, tenderness, and the formation of pus-filled lesions.

Gastrointestinal symptoms are also common with bacterial infections. These may include nausea, vomiting, diarrhea, and abdominal pain. In severe cases, the infection can lead to dehydration, which requires immediate medical attention.

Bacterial infections can also affect the urinary tract, causing symptoms such as frequent urination, pain or burning during urination, and cloudy or bloody urine. If you experience any of these symptoms, it is important to seek medical advice to prevent the infection from spreading to the kidneys.

In some cases, bacterial infections can lead to systemic symptoms, affecting the entire body. These may include rapid breathing, elevated heart rate, confusion, and even organ failure. Such systemic infections require emergency medical attention.

It is important to note that while these symptoms are generally associated with bacterial infections, they can also be caused by other types of infections or medical conditions. Therefore, it is essential to consult a healthcare professional for an accurate diagnosis and appropriate treatment.

As students interested in infectious diseases, being knowledgeable about the general symptoms of bacterial infections can help you make informed decisions about your health and the health of those around you. By recognizing these symptoms early on, you can seek appropriate medical care and contribute to the prevention and control of bacterial infectious diseases.

Remember, prevention is always better than cure. Maintaining good hygiene practices, such as regular handwashing and keeping your living spaces clean, can significantly reduce your risk of contracting bacterial infections. Stay informed, stay proactive, and prioritize your health and well-being.

Diagnostic Methods for Bacterial Infections

In the field of infectious diseases, accurate and timely diagnosis is crucial for effective treatment and prevention of bacterial infections. Diagnostic methods play a vital role in identifying the causative agent, determining the severity of the infection, and guiding appropriate treatment strategies. This subchapter explores the various diagnostic methods used in the identification and management of bacterial infections.

One of the most common diagnostic methods is the culture and sensitivity test. This involves collecting a sample from the infected area, such as blood, urine, or wound, and culturing it in a laboratory to isolate and identify the bacteria causing the infection. The isolated bacteria are then subjected to sensitivity testing to determine which antibiotics can effectively treat the infection. This method helps healthcare professionals select the most appropriate antibiotic therapy, preventing the misuse of antibiotics and the development of antibiotic resistance.

Another widely used diagnostic method is polymerase chain reaction (PCR). PCR enables the detection of bacterial DNA or RNA in patient samples, even in small quantities. By targeting specific genetic markers, PCR can identify the presence of the bacteria causing the infection rapidly and accurately. This method is particularly helpful in cases where traditional culture methods may be time-consuming or ineffective, such as in fastidious or slow-growing bacteria.

Immunological tests are also valuable diagnostic tools for bacterial infections. These tests detect the presence of specific antibodies or antigens in patient samples. For example, the enzyme-linked immunosorbent assay (ELISA) detects bacterial antigens or antibodies in blood samples, aiding in the diagnosis of infections like Lyme disease or Helicobacter pylori. Rapid antigen tests, such as the strep test, are commonly used in the diagnosis of streptococcal infections like strep throat.

In recent years, molecular techniques like next-generation sequencing (NGS) have revolutionized the field of bacterial diagnostics. NGS allows for the rapid and comprehensive analysis of bacterial genomes, enabling the identification of bacterial species, the detection of antibiotic resistance genes, and the tracking of bacterial outbreaks. This technique provides valuable insights into the transmission dynamics of bacterial infections, facilitating the implementation of effective infection control measures.

In conclusion, accurate and timely diagnosis is critical in the management of bacterial infections. By utilizing various diagnostic methods such as culture and sensitivity tests, PCR, immunological tests, and molecular techniques, healthcare professionals can accurately identify the causative agent and determine appropriate treatment strategies. Advancements in diagnostic methods continue to improve our ability to combat bacterial infections effectively, leading to better outcomes for patients.

Laboratory Tests for Bacterial Infections

When it comes to diagnosing bacterial infections, laboratory tests play a crucial role in providing accurate and reliable results. These tests help healthcare professionals identify the specific bacteria causing the infection, determine its susceptibility to antibiotics, and monitor the effectiveness of the treatment. In this subchapter, we will explore the different laboratory tests used in the diagnosis of bacterial infections.

1. Gram Stain: The Gram stain is a quick and inexpensive test that helps identify the bacterial species causing the infection. This test involves staining a sample of the patient's bodily fluid or tissue and observing it under a microscope. Bacteria can either be Gram-positive or Gram-negative, which provides valuable information for further diagnosis and treatment decisions.

2. Culture and Sensitivity: Culturing the bacteria from a patient's sample allows for their identification and susceptibility testing. By growing the bacteria in a controlled environment, healthcare professionals can determine the best antibiotic(s) to treat the infection effectively. This test may take a few days to yield results, but it provides critical information for targeted therapy.

3. Polymerase Chain Reaction (PCR): PCR is a molecular technique used to detect the presence of bacterial DNA in a patient's sample. This test is highly sensitive and specific, enabling the identification of bacteria that are difficult to culture or grow in the laboratory. PCR can rapidly diagnose bacterial infections, allowing for prompt initiation of appropriate treatment.

4. Serological Tests: Serological tests detect the antibodies produced by the immune system in response to a bacterial infection. These tests can determine if a person has been previously exposed to a specific bacterium or is currently infected. They are particularly useful for diagnosing bacterial infections that cannot be easily cultured or detected by other means.

5. Blood Tests: Blood tests, such as complete blood count (CBC) and C-reactive protein (CRP), are often used to assess the severity of a bacterial infection. CBC measures the number of white blood cells, which can indicate an ongoing infection, while CRP levels indicate inflammation in the body.

Understanding the different laboratory tests used to diagnose bacterial infections is essential for students studying infectious diseases. By learning about these tests, students can grasp the importance of accurate diagnosis and appropriate treatment. Remember, early and accurate identification of bacterial infections is crucial for providing timely and effective interventions, improving patient outcomes, and preventing the spread of these infections to others.

In conclusion, laboratory tests are invaluable tools in diagnosing bacterial infections. From Gram stains to serological tests, each test provides unique information that aids in the identification and treatment of bacterial infections. By familiarizing themselves with these tests, students can develop a comprehensive understanding of the diagnostic process and its significance in combating infectious diseases.

Chapter 6: Treatment and Management of Bacterial Infectious Diseases

Antibiotics and their Role in Treating Bacterial Infections

Introduction:
As students studying infectious diseases, it is crucial to have a clear understanding of antibiotics and their role in treating bacterial infections. Antibiotics are powerful medications that have revolutionized the field of medicine. They have saved countless lives and played a significant role in combating bacterial infections. In this subchapter, we will delve into the world of antibiotics, exploring their history, mechanisms of action, types, and the importance of responsible antibiotic use.

History of Antibiotics:
The discovery of antibiotics can be attributed to various scientists, with Alexander Fleming's accidental discovery of penicillin being a breakthrough moment. Since then, numerous antibiotics have been developed, each targeting specific bacteria and helping to alleviate the suffering caused by infectious diseases.

Mechanisms of Action:
Antibiotics work in different ways to combat bacterial infections. Some inhibit the ability of bacteria to form cell walls, rendering them vulnerable and unable to survive. Others disrupt essential bacterial metabolic processes or inhibit protein synthesis, ultimately leading to bacterial death. Understanding these mechanisms is vital in selecting the appropriate antibiotic for specific infections.

Types of Antibiotics:
There are several classes of antibiotics, each with its unique

properties and spectrum of activity. Broad-spectrum antibiotics, such as penicillin and tetracycline, can target a wide range of bacteria. On the other hand, narrow-spectrum antibiotics, like vancomycin, are effective against specific types of bacteria. It is important to note that antibiotics are ineffective against viral infections, such as the common cold or flu.

The Importance of Responsible Antibiotic Use: While antibiotics are powerful tools against bacterial infections, their misuse or overuse can lead to adverse consequences. The emergence of antibiotic resistance poses a significant threat to public health. It is crucial for students to understand the importance of responsible antibiotic use, including completing the prescribed course, not sharing antibiotics with others, and avoiding self-medication. Additionally, efforts to educate healthcare professionals and the general public about the appropriate use of antibiotics are key in preventing the spread of antibiotic-resistant bacteria.

Conclusion:
Antibiotics have played a vital role in the treatment of bacterial infections, saving countless lives and reducing morbidity. As students interested in infectious diseases, it is essential to have a comprehensive understanding of antibiotics, including their history, mechanisms of action, different types, and the importance of responsible antibiotic use. By utilizing antibiotics responsibly, we can ensure their continued effectiveness in combating bacterial infections and contribute to the global efforts in mitigating the threat of antibiotic resistance.

Vaccines for Bacterial Infections

Vaccines have revolutionized the field of medicine by providing effective prevention against various infectious diseases, including bacterial infections. In this subchapter, we will explore the importance of vaccines in combating bacterial infections and how they work to protect individuals from these diseases.

Bacterial infections pose a significant threat to public health, causing various diseases ranging from mild to severe. Fortunately, vaccines have been developed to prevent many bacterial infections, including those caused by pathogens like Streptococcus pneumoniae, Bordetella pertussis, and Neisseria meningitidis. These vaccines have proven to be highly effective in reducing the incidence and severity of these diseases, thus saving countless lives.

One of the most well-known vaccines for bacterial infections is the pneumococcal vaccine, which protects against pneumococcal disease, including pneumonia, meningitis, and bloodstream infections. This vaccine is recommended for all children and adults, particularly those at higher risk, such as the elderly and individuals with certain medical conditions.

Another crucial vaccine is the pertussis vaccine, which prevents whooping cough caused by Bordetella pertussis. Whooping cough can be particularly dangerous for infants and young children, making this vaccine an essential part of childhood immunization schedules.

Furthermore, the meningococcal vaccine protects against meningococcal disease, a severe infection that can cause meningitis and bloodstream infections. This vaccine is recommended for adolescents and young adults, as they are at higher risk of contracting this disease.

Vaccines for bacterial infections work by stimulating the immune system to produce a response against specific bacteria. They contain either killed bacteria or components of bacteria that cannot cause disease but can still trigger an immune response. When a person is vaccinated, their immune system recognizes these components as foreign and mounts a defense, producing antibodies that can recognize and neutralize the bacteria if they ever encounter it in the future.

It is important for students to understand the significance of vaccines in preventing bacterial infections. By getting vaccinated, individuals not only protect themselves but also contribute to the overall public health, as vaccinated individuals are less likely to transmit the bacteria to others. This concept, known as herd immunity, plays a crucial role in reducing the spread of infectious diseases within communities.

In conclusion, vaccines have played a pivotal role in the prevention and control of bacterial infections. By providing information on the importance of vaccines for bacterial infections, this subchapter aims to equip students with knowledge that will empower them to make informed decisions about their health and contribute to the fight against infectious diseases.

Prevention Strategies for Bacterial Infections

Bacterial infections are a common health concern that affects millions of people worldwide. These infections can range from mild to severe and can have significant consequences if left untreated. Fortunately, there are several effective prevention strategies that can help students reduce their risk of bacterial infections and maintain a healthy lifestyle.

1. Personal Hygiene: Proper personal hygiene practices play a crucial role in preventing the spread of bacterial infections. Students should make it a habit to wash their hands regularly with soap and water, especially before eating, after using the restroom, and after coming into contact with potentially contaminated surfaces.

2. Vaccination: Vaccines are a powerful tool in preventing bacterial infections. Students should ensure they are up-to-date with their immunizations, including those for common bacterial infections like tetanus, diphtheria, pertussis, and meningococcal disease. Vaccination not only protects the individual but also helps prevent the spread of infections within the community.

3. Food Safety: Bacterial infections can be transmitted through contaminated food and water. Students should practice good food safety measures, such as properly storing and cooking food, avoiding cross-contamination, and consuming only pasteurized dairy products. Additionally, it is important to drink clean and safe water and avoid consuming raw or undercooked meats, seafood, and eggs.

4. Respiratory Etiquette: Bacterial infections can be transmitted through respiratory droplets when an infected

person coughs or sneezes. Students should cover their mouth and nose with a tissue or their elbow when coughing or sneezing, and dispose of tissues properly. Avoiding close contact with individuals who have respiratory infections can also help prevent the spread of bacteria.

5. Environmental Cleanliness: Keeping the environment clean and disinfected can help reduce the risk of bacterial infections. Students should regularly clean frequently touched surfaces, such as doorknobs, desks, and shared electronic devices. Additionally, avoiding sharing personal items like towels, utensils, and water bottles can help prevent the transmission of bacteria.

6. Safe Sex Practices: Certain bacterial infections, such as chlamydia, gonorrhea, and syphilis, can be sexually transmitted. Students should practice safe sex by using barrier methods, such as condoms, and getting regular screenings for sexually transmitted infections.

By adopting these prevention strategies, students can significantly reduce their risk of bacterial infections and maintain good overall health. It is important to remember that prevention is always better than cure, and being proactive in protecting oneself and others from bacterial infections is a responsible and essential practice for students in the field of infectious diseases.

Chapter 7: Antibiotic Resistance in Bacterial Infectious Diseases

Understanding Antibiotic Resistance

Antibiotic resistance is a growing concern in the field of infectious diseases. As students studying bacterial infectious diseases, it is crucial for us to comprehend this phenomenon and its implications. This subchapter aims to provide a comprehensive understanding of antibiotic resistance, including its causes, mechanisms, and potential consequences.

Antibiotics are powerful medications used to treat bacterial infections. They work by either killing the bacteria or inhibiting their growth, allowing the immune system to effectively eliminate the infection. However, over time, bacteria can develop resistance to these drugs, rendering them ineffective. This resistance arises due to various factors, such as overuse and misuse of antibiotics, inadequate dosing, and incomplete treatment courses.

The mechanisms behind antibiotic resistance are diverse and complex. Bacteria can acquire resistance through genetic mutations or by obtaining resistance genes from other bacteria through horizontal gene transfer. These resistance genes often encode enzymes that inactivate antibiotics, alter drug targets, or pump out the drugs from inside the bacterial cells. As a result, bacteria become unaffected by the antibiotics, leading to treatment failure.

The consequences of antibiotic resistance are significant. It can prolong the duration of infections, increase the severity of symptoms, and even result in life-threatening complications. Additionally, resistant bacteria can spread from person to person, posing a threat to public health. If left unchecked, antibiotic resistance could potentially lead to a post-antibiotic era, where even minor infections become untreatable, jeopardizing medical advancements and increasing mortality rates.

To combat antibiotic resistance, it is essential for us as students to adopt responsible antibiotic use practices. This includes taking antibiotics only when prescribed by a healthcare professional, completing the full course of treatment, and never sharing or using leftover antibiotics. Additionally, we must advocate for improved infection prevention and control measures, such as proper hand hygiene and vaccination, to reduce the need for antibiotics.

In conclusion, understanding antibiotic resistance is crucial for students studying bacterial infectious diseases. We must grasp the causes, mechanisms, and consequences of resistance to effectively combat this global health threat. By practicing responsible antibiotic use and advocating for infection prevention, we can contribute to preserving the efficacy of antibiotics and safeguarding public health for future generations.

Factors Contributing to Antibiotic Resistance

Introduction:
Antibiotic resistance is a growing concern in the field of infectious diseases. As students studying bacterial infectious diseases, it is crucial to understand the factors that contribute to this phenomenon. This subchapter will delve into the key factors that drive antibiotic resistance, providing you with a comprehensive understanding of this global health issue.

1. Overuse and Misuse of Antibiotics:
One of the leading factors contributing to antibiotic resistance is the overuse and misuse of these medications. Students must understand that antibiotics are only effective against bacterial infections, not viral infections like the common cold or flu. Overprescribing antibiotics and patient non-compliance with prescribed dosages can lead to the development of antibiotic-resistant bacteria.

2. Agricultural Practices:
Another significant factor is the use of antibiotics in agriculture. Antibiotics are commonly given to livestock to promote growth and prevent disease. However, the widespread use of antibiotics in animal farming contributes to the emergence of antibiotic-resistant bacteria that can be transferred to humans through the food chain.

3. Inadequate Infection Control:
Poor infection control practices in healthcare settings can also contribute to antibiotic resistance. Students should be aware of the importance of proper hand hygiene, sterilization of medical equipment, and adherence to guidelines for preventing the spread of infections. Failure to implement these measures can

lead to the transmission of antibiotic-resistant bacteria among patients.

4. Lack of New Antibiotics: The development of new antibiotics has significantly slowed down in recent years. Pharmaceutical companies face financial challenges and regulatory hurdles in bringing new antibiotics to market. This limited arsenal of antibiotics allows bacteria to evolve and become resistant to existing medications.

5. Global Travel and Migration: The ease and frequency of global travel facilitate the spread of antibiotic-resistant bacteria across countries. Students should understand the role of international travel and migration in the dissemination of resistant strains and the need for global collaboration to address this challenge.

Conclusion:
Understanding the factors contributing to antibiotic resistance is crucial for students studying infectious diseases. Overuse and misuse of antibiotics, agricultural practices, inadequate infection control, lack of new antibiotics, and global travel all play significant roles. By recognizing these factors and taking appropriate measures, students can contribute to the efforts aimed at combating antibiotic resistance, ensuring the effectiveness of antibiotics for future generations.

Impact of Antibiotic Resistance on Bacterial Infections

In recent years, the rise of antibiotic resistance has become a major concern in the field of infectious diseases. Antibiotic resistance refers to the ability of bacteria to survive and multiply in the presence of antibiotics that were previously effective in killing them. This phenomenon has created significant challenges for healthcare professionals and has led to a global crisis in the treatment of bacterial infections.

The impact of antibiotic resistance on bacterial infections cannot be overstated. Previously treatable infections, such as pneumonia, urinary tract infections, and skin infections, are now becoming more difficult to manage. This means that patients may experience prolonged illness, increased hospitalizations, and even death. The development of antibiotic resistance not only affects individual patients but also has broader societal consequences. The economic burden of antibiotic-resistant infections is substantial, with increased healthcare costs and loss of productivity.

One of the main causes of antibiotic resistance is the misuse and overuse of antibiotics. Students should be aware of the importance of using antibiotics only when necessary and as prescribed by a healthcare professional. Taking antibiotics for viral infections, such as the common cold or the flu, is ineffective and contributes to the development of resistance. It is crucial to educate the general public about the appropriate use of antibiotics to help combat the spread of antibiotic resistance.

Furthermore, students should understand that antibiotic resistance is not limited to humans. The use of antibiotics in agriculture, particularly in livestock farming, has also contributed to the emergence of resistant bacteria. Consuming food contaminated with antibiotic-resistant bacteria can lead to infections that are difficult to treat. By advocating for responsible antibiotic use in both healthcare and agricultural settings, students can contribute to the prevention and control of antibiotic resistance.

In conclusion, the impact of antibiotic resistance on bacterial infections is a significant concern in the field of infectious diseases. Students should be aware of the consequences of antibiotic resistance, both at an individual and societal level. By understanding the importance of responsible antibiotic use and advocating for appropriate practices, students can play a crucial role in combating this global health crisis. It is essential for the future generation to be well-informed and proactive in the fight against antibiotic resistance to ensure effective treatment options for bacterial infections.

Chapter 8: Emerging Bacterial Infectious Diseases

Methicillin-Resistant Staphylococcus aureus (MRSA)

Introduction:
In recent years, infectious diseases have become a major concern worldwide. One such infection that has gained attention is Methicillin-Resistant Staphylococcus aureus (MRSA). This subchapter aims to provide students with a comprehensive understanding of MRSA, including its causes, symptoms, and treatments.

Understanding MRSA:
Staphylococcus aureus is a common bacterium that can be found on the skin and in the respiratory tract of healthy individuals. However, some strains of this bacterium have evolved resistance to methicillin, an antibiotic commonly used to treat staph infections. This resistance makes MRSA a formidable pathogen.

Causes and Transmission:
MRSA can be acquired through direct skin-to-skin contact with an infected person or by touching contaminated surfaces. It often affects individuals with weakened immune systems, such as hospital patients, athletes, and individuals living in crowded conditions. Poor hygiene practices, such as sharing personal items or not washing hands properly, can also increase the risk of MRSA transmission.

Symptoms:
MRSA infections can present in different forms, ranging from minor skin infections to life-threatening conditions. Common symptoms include redness, swelling, and warmth around the site of infection, accompanied by pain or pus-filled abscesses.

It is essential to seek medical attention promptly if any signs of infection appear.

Treatment:
The treatment of MRSA infections can be challenging due to antibiotic resistance. Healthcare providers typically rely on a combination of antibiotics to combat MRSA effectively. In severe cases, hospitalization and intravenous antibiotics may be necessary. Prevention is crucial to reduce the spread of MRSA, and it includes practicing good hygiene, avoiding close contact with infected individuals, and keeping wounds clean and covered.

Preventing MRSA Infections:
To prevent MRSA infections, students should adopt simple yet effective measures. Regular handwashing with soap and water for at least 20 seconds is crucial. Avoiding sharing personal items, such as towels, razors, and clothing, can also minimize the risk of transmission. Cleaning and disinfecting frequently-touched surfaces, such as doorknobs and cell phones, is another preventive measure that students should practice.

Conclusion:
Methicillin-Resistant Staphylococcus aureus (MRSA) is a concerning bacterial infection that poses a threat to public health. Understanding the causes, symptoms, and treatments of MRSA is essential for students interested in infectious diseases. By promoting good hygiene practices and taking preventive measures, students can contribute to the prevention and control of MRSA infections in their communities.

Clostridioides difficile Infections

Clostridioides difficile, commonly known as C. difficile, is a bacterium that causes a variety of symptoms ranging from mild diarrhea to life-threatening inflammation of the colon. This bacterium is commonly found in the environment, especially in healthcare settings such as hospitals and long-term care facilities. In recent years, C. difficile infections have become a major concern due to their increasing prevalence and resistance to antibiotics.

C. difficile infections occur when the bacterium overgrows in the intestines, usually as a result of disruption in the normal gut flora. This disruption can be caused by the use of certain antibiotics, which kill off the beneficial bacteria in the gut that normally keep C. difficile in check. Other risk factors for C. difficile infections include advanced age, underlying medical conditions, and prolonged hospital stays.

The symptoms of C. difficile infections can vary widely, but the most common one is diarrhea. Other symptoms may include abdominal pain, fever, loss of appetite, and nausea. In severe cases, the infection can progress to a condition called pseudomembranous colitis, which is characterized by severe inflammation of the colon and can be life-threatening if not promptly treated.

Diagnosing C. difficile infections involves testing a stool sample for the presence of the bacterium's toxins. This can be done using various laboratory techniques, including enzyme immunoassays and polymerase chain reaction (PCR) assays. Prompt and accurate diagnosis is crucial for appropriate treatment and preventing the spread of the infection.

Treatment of C. difficile infections typically involves stopping the use of the offending antibiotics and administering specific antibiotics that target the bacterium. In some cases, more aggressive interventions may be necessary, such as fecal microbiota transplantation, which involves transferring healthy bacteria from a donor into the patient's colon to restore the balance of gut flora.

Preventing C. difficile infections is a multifaceted approach that includes strict adherence to infection control practices in healthcare settings, such as hand hygiene and appropriate use of antibiotics. Students pursuing careers in healthcare or those interested in infectious diseases should be aware of the risk factors, symptoms, and preventive measures associated with C. difficile infections.

In conclusion, Clostridioides difficile infections are a significant concern in healthcare settings and can cause a range of symptoms from mild to severe. Prompt diagnosis and appropriate treatment are vital to prevent complications and reduce the spread of the infection. By understanding the risk factors and practicing good infection control measures, students can contribute to the prevention and management of C. difficile infections in the future.

Carbapenem-Resistant Enterobacteriaceae (CRE)

Carbapenem-Resistant Enterobacteriaceae (CRE): A Growing Concern in Infectious Diseases

In recent years, the rise of antibiotic resistance has become a major global health concern. One particular group of bacteria that has garnered attention is Carbapenem-Resistant Enterobacteriaceae, commonly known as CRE. This subchapter aims to provide students with a comprehensive understanding of CRE, including its causes, symptoms, and available treatments.

CRE is a type of bacteria that belongs to the Enterobacteriaceae family, which includes well-known pathogens such as Escherichia coli and Klebsiella pneumoniae. These bacteria are normally found in the human gut, but when they become resistant to carbapenem antibiotics, they can cause severe infections, often resulting in high mortality rates.

The main cause of CRE is the acquisition of certain genes that produce enzymes called carbapenemases. These enzymes can break down carbapenem antibiotics, rendering them ineffective. CRE can be acquired through various means, including healthcare-associated infections, community-acquired infections, and even through contact with contaminated surfaces or food.

Symptoms of CRE infections vary depending on the site of infection. Common manifestations include urinary tract infections, bloodstream infections, pneumonia, and intra-abdominal infections. In severe cases, CRE infections can lead to sepsis, a life-threatening condition.

Treating CRE infections poses a significant challenge due to limited treatment options. Carbapenems are considered the drugs of choice for Enterobacteriaceae infections, but since CRE is resistant to these antibiotics, alternative treatment strategies must be employed. These include using combination therapy with multiple antibiotics or resorting to older, less effective antibiotics that may have more side effects.

Preventing the spread of CRE is crucial to combat its increasing prevalence. Students should be aware of the importance of hand hygiene, proper infection control practices, and the appropriate use of antibiotics. It is equally essential to raise awareness among healthcare professionals and policymakers to implement strategies such as surveillance, early detection, and prudent use of antibiotics to curb the spread of CRE.

In conclusion, Carbapenem-Resistant Enterobacteriaceae is a growing concern in the field of infectious diseases. Students must understand the causes, symptoms, and treatment options available for these infections. By promoting awareness and implementing preventive measures, we can collectively work towards reducing the burden of CRE and safeguarding the effectiveness of antibiotics for future generations.

Chapter 9: Case Studies: Real-Life Examples of Bacterial Infectious Diseases

Tuberculosis Outbreak in a Community

Tuberculosis (TB) is a highly contagious bacterial infectious disease caused by Mycobacterium tuberculosis. It primarily affects the respiratory system but can also spread to other parts of the body. In recent years, there has been a concerning rise in the number of TB cases worldwide, leading to outbreaks in several communities. This subchapter aims to provide students with a comprehensive understanding of the causes, symptoms, and treatments of TB, as well as the measures to prevent and control its spread.

Causes of Tuberculosis Outbreaks: TB outbreaks occur when the disease spreads rapidly within a community. Factors contributing to such outbreaks include overcrowded living conditions, poor ventilation, inadequate access to healthcare facilities, and the presence of drug-resistant strains of the bacteria. Students need to be aware of these factors and understand how they contribute to the emergence and spread of TB in their communities.

Symptoms of Tuberculosis: Recognizing the symptoms of TB is crucial for early detection and treatment. Common symptoms include persistent coughing, chest pain, weight loss, fatigue, and night sweats. Students should be aware that TB can also affect other parts of the body, such as the bones, joints, and kidneys, leading to different sets of symptoms. By being knowledgeable about these symptoms, students can help identify potential TB cases and encourage affected individuals to seek medical assistance promptly.

Treatment and Prevention:
Treating TB requires a combination of antibiotics over an extended period. It is essential for students to understand the importance of completing the full course of treatment to prevent drug resistance and relapse. Additionally, preventive measures such as vaccination (BCG) and proper hygiene practices can significantly reduce the risk of contracting and spreading the disease. Students should be encouraged to maintain good respiratory hygiene, such as covering their mouths when coughing or sneezing, and to avoid close contact with individuals displaying TB symptoms.

Community Involvement:
Students have a vital role to play in preventing and controlling TB outbreaks within their communities. By raising awareness, promoting healthy habits, and advocating for improved healthcare facilities, students can contribute to the overall well-being of their communities. Collaboration with local health authorities and organizations can also provide students with opportunities to engage in community outreach programs, such as organizing educational campaigns and facilitating screenings for early detection.

In conclusion, understanding the causes, symptoms, and treatments of tuberculosis is crucial for students interested in infectious diseases. By familiarizing themselves with these aspects and actively participating in preventive measures, students can play a significant role in preventing and controlling TB outbreaks within their communities.

Contamination of Food with Salmonella

Foodborne illnesses are a significant concern worldwide, affecting millions of people each year. One of the most common culprits behind these infections is Salmonella, a bacteria that can contaminate various types of food. This subchapter delves into the contamination of food with Salmonella, providing students with essential knowledge about this infectious disease.

Salmonella is a type of bacteria that can cause salmonellosis, a foodborne illness characterized by symptoms such as diarrhea, abdominal pain, fever, and vomiting. It is primarily transmitted through the consumption of contaminated food, especially raw or undercooked meat, poultry, eggs, and unpasteurized dairy products. Additionally, fruits, vegetables, and spices can also become contaminated if they come into contact with animal feces or contaminated water during production or processing.

Understanding the sources of Salmonella contamination is crucial in preventing the spread of this bacteria. Students need to be aware that poor food handling practices, such as improper storage temperatures and inadequate cooking or reheating, can contribute to the proliferation of Salmonella in food. Cross-contamination, where raw and cooked food come into contact with each other, is another common cause of foodborne illnesses.

To prevent the contamination of food with Salmonella, students should practice good food hygiene habits. This includes washing hands thoroughly before and after handling food, using separate cutting boards for raw and cooked foods, and cooking food to the appropriate internal temperature. It is essential to avoid consuming raw or undercooked eggs, meat, and poultry, as these are more likely to harbor Salmonella.

In the event of a suspected Salmonella infection, it is crucial for students to seek medical attention promptly. Most cases of salmonellosis resolve on their own within a week, but severe cases may require medical intervention. Dehydration is a common complication of this illness, so staying hydrated is essential.

With the knowledge gained from this subchapter, students can become proactive in preventing the contamination of food with Salmonella. By adopting good food hygiene practices and being vigilant about the sources of contamination, they can protect themselves and others from this common foodborne illness.

Hospital-Acquired Infections: Case of MRSA

In a healthcare setting, patients come seeking treatment and care, but unfortunately, they can also be vulnerable to acquiring infections. One such infection that often spreads within hospitals is Methicillin-Resistant Staphylococcus aureus, commonly known as MRSA. As students studying infectious diseases, it is crucial for us to understand the causes, symptoms, and treatments of this particular hospital-acquired infection.

MRSA is a type of bacteria that is resistant to many antibiotics, making it difficult to treat. It is commonly found on the skin or in the nose of healthy individuals, but it can cause infections when it enters the body through an open wound, surgical site, or invasive medical devices like catheters. Once inside the body, MRSA can cause a range of infections, from mild skin infections to life-threatening bloodstream infections and pneumonia.

The symptoms of MRSA may vary depending on the site of infection. Skin infections often present as red, swollen, and painful sores or boils. These can be accompanied by fever and chills. In more severe cases, MRSA can cause pneumonia, which leads to symptoms such as difficulty breathing, chest pain, and a high fever.

Preventing the spread of MRSA requires strict adherence to infection control practices. Healthcare professionals must practice good hand hygiene, wearing gloves and gowns when necessary, and using proper disinfection techniques. Patients can also play a role by practicing good personal hygiene, such as regular handwashing and keeping wounds clean and covered.

Treatment for MRSA infections may involve a combination of antibiotics, as some strains have developed resistance to multiple drugs. In severe cases, hospitalization may be required for intravenous antibiotics. It is essential to complete the full course of antibiotics as prescribed, even if the symptoms improve, to ensure complete eradication of the bacteria.

As students interested in infectious diseases, it is important to be aware of the risks and preventive measures associated with hospital-acquired infections like MRSA. By practicing good hygiene and understanding the importance of infection control, we can contribute to reducing the spread of MRSA and other similar infections in healthcare settings.

In conclusion, MRSA is a significant concern in hospitals, causing infections that range from mild to life-threatening. Understanding the causes, symptoms, and treatments of MRSA is vital for students studying infectious diseases. By promoting good hygiene practices and adhering to infection control protocols, we can help prevent the spread of MRSA and protect both patients and healthcare workers from this hospital-acquired infection.

Chapter 10: Future Perspectives in Bacterial Infectious Diseases

Advancements in Bacterial Infection Research

In recent years, there have been significant advancements in the field of bacterial infection research, leading to a greater understanding of the causes, symptoms, and treatments of these diseases. This subchapter explores some of the key breakthroughs and their implications for students studying infectious diseases.

One major area of progress is in the identification and classification of bacterial strains. DNA sequencing technologies have revolutionized the way scientists analyze bacterial genomes, allowing for the identification of specific strains and the tracking of their spread. This has been particularly valuable in outbreaks and epidemics, as it enables researchers to quickly determine the source of infection and implement appropriate control measures.

Furthermore, advancements in molecular biology have led to a better understanding of the mechanisms by which bacteria cause infections. Scientists have discovered new virulence factors and pathways that bacteria use to invade host cells and evade the immune system. This knowledge has opened up new possibilities for developing targeted therapies and vaccines that can disrupt these processes and prevent or treat bacterial infections more effectively.

Another area of advancement is the development of novel diagnostic techniques. Traditional methods of bacterial identification, such as culturing and microscopy, are time-consuming and often unreliable. However, new molecular-based techniques, such as polymerase chain reaction (PCR) and next-generation sequencing, have greatly improved the speed and accuracy of bacterial diagnosis. These techniques can detect bacterial DNA or RNA directly from patient samples, allowing for rapid and precise identification of the infecting organism.

In terms of treatment, the rise of antibiotic resistance has posed a significant challenge. However, research into alternative strategies has yielded promising results. For example, bacteriophages, which are viruses that infect and kill bacteria, have shown potential as a targeted therapy for bacterial infections. Additionally, the use of bacteriocins, naturally occurring antimicrobial peptides produced by bacteria, is being explored as a potential alternative to traditional antibiotics.

Overall, the advancements in bacterial infection research have provided students studying infectious diseases with a wealth of new knowledge and opportunities. By understanding the mechanisms of bacterial infections and the strategies employed by bacteria to cause disease, students can contribute to the development of innovative diagnostic tools, therapeutic approaches, and preventive measures. As the field continues to evolve, it is crucial for students to stay up-to-date with the latest research findings and collaborate with other experts to combat the ever-evolving threat of bacterial infections.

Potential Solutions for Antibiotic Resistance

In recent years, the rise of antibiotic resistance has become a major concern in the field of infectious diseases. Bacteria have evolved and developed resistance mechanisms, making many antibiotics less effective in treating infections. This subchapter explores potential solutions for antibiotic resistance, providing students with valuable insights into the current strategies being employed to combat this global threat.

1. Antibiotic Stewardship Programs: One of the most effective ways to address antibiotic resistance is through antibiotic stewardship programs. These programs aim to promote the appropriate use of antibiotics by educating healthcare professionals and the public about the importance of responsible antibiotic use. By ensuring that antibiotics are only prescribed when necessary and following the recommended dosage and duration, we can minimize the development of resistance.

2. Development of New Antibiotics: Another crucial aspect in the fight against antibiotic resistance is the development of new antibiotics. Researchers are constantly exploring new avenues to discover novel compounds that can effectively combat drug-resistant bacteria. Students interested in microbiology and pharmaceutical sciences can contribute to this field by pursuing research and innovation in antibiotic development.

3. Combination Therapies: Combination therapies involve using multiple antibiotics simultaneously or in sequence to overcome resistance mechanisms employed by bacteria. This approach can enhance the effectiveness of existing antibiotics and prevent the

emergence of resistance. Students studying medicine or pharmacology can explore the potential of combination therapies to combat antibiotic resistance.

4. Bacteriophage Therapy: Bacteriophage therapy is an emerging field that utilizes bacteriophages, which are viruses that infect and kill bacteria, as an alternative to antibiotics. Bacteriophages are highly specific in targeting bacteria, reducing the risk of resistance development. Students interested in virology and molecular biology can explore the potential of bacteriophage therapy as a solution for antibiotic resistance.

5. Public Awareness and Education: Lastly, raising public awareness about antibiotic resistance is crucial in combating this issue. Students can play an active role in educating their peers, families, and communities about the responsible use of antibiotics, the consequences of misuse, and the importance of completing prescribed courses. This awareness can help reduce unnecessary antibiotic use and slow down the development of resistance.

In conclusion, addressing antibiotic resistance requires a multi-faceted approach. By implementing antibiotic stewardship programs, developing new antibiotics, exploring combination therapies, researching bacteriophage therapy, and raising public awareness, we can work towards mitigating the impact of antibiotic resistance and preserving the effectiveness of these life-saving drugs. As students, you have the potential to contribute to these efforts and make a positive impact in the field of infectious diseases.

Importance of Public Health Education and Awareness

In today's interconnected world, public health education and awareness play a crucial role in combating infectious diseases. As students pursuing knowledge in the field of infectious diseases, it is essential to understand the significance of public health education and how it can positively impact our lives and the broader community.

Firstly, public health education raises awareness about the causes, symptoms, and treatments of bacterial infectious diseases. By disseminating accurate information to the public, it helps individuals understand the risks associated with various pathogens and empowers them to take necessary precautions. This knowledge is particularly important for students as they often find themselves in close proximity with others in schools, universities, and dormitories. By learning about infectious diseases, students can adopt healthy habits and preventive measures such as proper hand hygiene, vaccination, and safe food handling practices, reducing the risk of transmission within their communities.

Moreover, public health education fosters a sense of responsibility and community engagement. When students are educated about the impact of their actions on public health, they become more conscious of their behavior and its consequences. They are more likely to practice good personal hygiene, adopt healthy lifestyles, and adhere to recommended vaccination schedules. By doing so, they not only protect themselves but also contribute to the well-being of their classmates, families, and society as a whole.

Public health education also promotes early detection and prompt treatment. When individuals are aware of the symptoms of bacterial infectious diseases, they are more likely to seek medical help at the earliest signs. This proactive approach leads to early diagnosis and timely treatment, preventing the spread of the disease and potentially saving lives. Students who possess this knowledge can identify symptoms in themselves or their peers and encourage seeking medical attention, thereby playing an active role in disease management and prevention.

Furthermore, public health education provides an understanding of the importance of vaccination programs. Students learn about the benefits of vaccines, including their role in preventing the spread of infectious diseases and protecting vulnerable populations. By being aware of the latest vaccination recommendations, students can ensure they are up to date with their immunizations, reducing the risk of contracting and transmitting diseases such as influenza, measles, and hepatitis.

In conclusion, public health education and awareness are vital tools in the fight against bacterial infectious diseases. As students in the field of infectious diseases, it is our responsibility to educate ourselves and others about the causes, symptoms, and treatments of these diseases. By promoting public health education, we empower individuals to make informed decisions, adopt preventive measures, and contribute to a healthier and safer community. Through our collective efforts, we can create a world where infectious diseases are better understood and effectively managed, ensuring the well-being of all.

Chapter 11: Conclusion and Resources

Summary of Key Points

In this subchapter, we will provide a concise overview of the key points discussed in the book "The Student's Handbook on Bacterial Infectious Diseases: Causes, Symptoms, and Treatments." This summary aims to provide students with a comprehensive understanding of the fundamental concepts related to infectious diseases caused by bacteria.

The book begins by introducing the basics of bacterial infections, focusing on the causes, symptoms, and transmission methods. It highlights the importance of personal hygiene, such as frequent handwashing, to prevent the spread of bacteria. Additionally, it emphasizes the significance of vaccination as a preventive measure against bacterial infections.

Next, the book delves into the various types of bacterial infectious diseases, including respiratory infections, gastrointestinal infections, skin infections, and urinary tract infections. Each section provides detailed information on the specific bacteria responsible for these diseases, their modes of transmission, and the common symptoms experienced by affected individuals.

Furthermore, the book explores the principles of bacterial diagnosis and laboratory testing. It educates students on the different techniques used to identify and confirm the presence of bacterial infections. It also emphasizes the significance of early diagnosis in initiating appropriate treatment and preventing the further spread of the infection.

The treatment section of the book offers insights into the various treatment options available for bacterial infections. It discusses the use of antibiotics, their mechanisms of action, and the importance of completing the full course of medication to prevent antibiotic resistance. The book also highlights the role of supportive care, such as rest, hydration, and pain relief, in managing bacterial infections effectively.

Lastly, the book addresses the importance of antibiotic stewardship and the global concern of antibiotic resistance. It educates students on the responsible use of antibiotics to minimize the development of drug-resistant bacteria. It also emphasizes the need for ongoing research and development of new antibiotics to combat emerging bacterial threats.

By summarizing these key points, the subchapter aims to provide students with a solid foundation in understanding bacterial infectious diseases. It equips them with essential knowledge to protect themselves and others from these infections, contribute to public health, and consider potential career paths in the field of infectious diseases.

Additional Resources for Further Reading

As a student delving into the fascinating field of infectious diseases, it is crucial to expand your knowledge beyond the content covered in this handbook. The world of bacterial infectious diseases is vast and constantly evolving, and to truly grasp the subject, it is essential to explore additional resources. This subchapter provides a list of valuable resources that will serve as a solid foundation for further reading and research.

1. Textbooks: To delve deeper into the causes, symptoms, and treatments of bacterial infectious diseases, textbooks are an excellent resource. Some highly recommended textbooks include "Principles of Bacteriology and Immunity" by Frank M. Burnet, "Medical Microbiology" by Patrick R. Murray, and "Mandell, Douglas, and Bennett's Principles and Practice of Infectious Diseases" by John E. Bennett. These comprehensive texts cover a wide range of bacterial infections and provide in-depth knowledge on the subject.

2. Academic Journals: Keeping up with the latest research is crucial in understanding the ever-changing landscape of bacterial infectious diseases. Academic journals such as "The Journal of Infectious Diseases," "Clinical Infectious Diseases," and "Emerging Infectious Diseases" publish cutting-edge research articles, case studies, and reviews. These journals will keep you updated on the latest breakthroughs and provide valuable insights from leading experts in the field.

3. Websites and Online Resources: The internet is a treasure trove of information, and several websites offer valuable resources on bacterial infectious diseases. The Centers for Disease Control and Prevention (CDC) and the World Health Organization (WHO) websites are excellent starting points for

reliable and up-to-date information on infectious diseases. Additionally, websites like Medscape, Mayo Clinic, and WebMD provide comprehensive articles, videos, and interactive tools to deepen your understanding.

4. Online Courses and Webinars: Many educational platforms offer online courses and webinars specifically focused on infectious diseases. Websites like Coursera, edX, and Khan Academy offer a variety of courses taught by renowned experts in the field. These courses allow you to learn at your own pace and provide a more interactive learning experience.

5. Professional Associations and Conferences: Joining professional associations related to infectious diseases, such as the Infectious Diseases Society of America (IDSA) or the European Society of Clinical Microbiology and Infectious Diseases (ESCMID), can provide access to a wealth of resources. These associations often organize conferences, webinars, and workshops where you can learn from leading experts and network with professionals in the field.

By utilizing these additional resources, you will enhance your understanding of bacterial infectious diseases and stay informed about the latest advancements. Remember, learning is a lifelong process, and the more you explore, the more equipped you will be to make a significant impact in the field of infectious diseases.

Glossary of Terms

In the realm of infectious diseases, it is essential to familiarize ourselves with the terminology commonly used in this field. This glossary aims to provide students with a comprehensive understanding of key terms related to bacterial infectious diseases, including their causes, symptoms, and treatments. By grasping these fundamental concepts, students can better navigate the complex world of infectious diseases and contribute to the advancement of medical knowledge.

1. Bacteria: Microscopic organisms that can cause infections. They are single-celled and can be either beneficial or harmful to humans.

2. Pathogen: A type of microorganism, such as bacteria, viruses, or fungi, that can cause disease.

3. Antibiotics: Medications used to treat bacterial infections by killing or inhibiting the growth of bacteria.

4. Resistance: The ability of bacteria to withstand the effects of antibiotics, making them less effective in treating infections.

5. Virulence: The degree of pathogenicity or the ability of a microorganism to cause disease.

6. Transmission: The process by which infectious diseases are spread from one individual to another, either through direct or indirect contact.

7. Outbreak: The occurrence of cases of a particular infectious disease in a community or region, often exceeding the usual number of cases.

8. Epidemic: A widespread outbreak of an infectious disease that affects a large number of people within a specific population or region.

9. Pandemic: A global outbreak of an infectious disease that affects multiple countries or continents.

10. Symptoms: Physical or psychological changes that indicate the presence of a disease, such as fever, cough, or fatigue.

11. Diagnosis: The process of identifying a disease or condition by considering the patient's symptoms, medical history, and diagnostic tests.

12. Treatment: The medical interventions employed to alleviate or cure a disease, which can include medication, surgery, or lifestyle modifications.

13. Vaccination: The administration of a vaccine to stimulate the immune system's production of antibodies against a specific infectious disease.

14. Immunity: The body's ability to resist or fight off an infectious disease due to previous exposure or vaccination.

15. Hygiene: Practices that promote cleanliness and prevent the spread of infectious diseases, such as handwashing, proper food handling, and sanitation.

By familiarizing themselves with these terms, students can better understand the causes, symptoms, and treatments of bacterial infectious diseases. This knowledge will empower them to make informed decisions about their health, contribute to the prevention of disease transmission, and potentially pursue careers in the field of infectious diseases.

Printed in the USA
CPSIA information can be obtained
at www.ICGtesting.com
LVHW012115230524
781044LV00013B/700